MEDICAL MISADVENTURE
…a sufferers account and the fallout after…

SEMISI PONE
BSc, MSc (Hons)

CONTENTS

INTRODUCTION

I decided to write this book, after 20 years of suffering from a vaccine injury, in the hope that it will help others in the same predicament. I know there has been increasing outcry from families of sufferers over vaccine injury, all over the world, but there is a kind of wanton inaction on the part of the Health Industry in New Zealand and other countries. It probably has more to do with business protection and reputation of companies producing the vaccine because any doubts over their vaccines will kill their businesses. The politicians who also deal with these issues are often fully aware of the consequences for the businesses and the Government of any large payouts over claims regarding vaccine injury or deaths.

We all accept that vaccines are very, very important tools in the fight against disease and protection of human health, and we also know that injuries to a small percent of patients/clients do occur.

What needs to happen, in my view, is that the Health Industry should have some mitigating contingency plans to deal with the small percentage of patients/clients who do get injured by the vaccines that were designed to protect them. We all differ in genetic makeup and sometimes the reaction of the immune system, for example, causes problems for the individuals who receive the vaccine. In my case, about 20 years now from the time I received the vaccine.

This book is an account of what I have noticed with my body over those 20 years. Hopefully, the scientists who do the research and development of those vaccines can use my account in their research and also the patients and sufferers in their search for some comfort.

CHAPTER 1. My background

I was born in the Kingdom of Tonga on the 11 of December 1961. I have been very healthy since birth and even though I have suffered from the normal barrage of diseases expected to affect children in the Kingdom of Tonga, a South Pacific Island, I was otherwise fine.

My Name

My birth name is Semisi Pule. I also added Pone at the end in 1977 when I sat my Tonga Higher Leaving Certificate. I continued using Semisi Pule Pone when I sat the New Zealand School Certificate, University Entrance Exams and at the University of Auckland. My father had added the SPPone to my birth certificate and passport in 1980 before I came to New Zealand so I can use both names legally. My father had to sign a sworn statement in the High Court of the

Kingdom of Tonga so I can use both names. The name on the passport and birth certificates was Semisi Pule also known as (aka) Semisi Pule Pone. From then on I used the short form Semisi Pone, which is the first and last names.

Why did I add Pone at the end of my name?

Just before I sat my Tonga Higher Leaving Certificate Exam, in 1977, I had noticed that my father was using the name Samisoni Pone and he never use the surname Pule. I suspect that perhaps he was proud of his father, whose 'shortname' was Pone. Everyone called him Pone even though his full name was Viliami Ponepate Pule. He was a Police Magistrate. I reasoned, as a 16 year old, that it would be strange for my name to be announced on the radio, if my examination is successful, as Semisi Pule when my father's name is Samisoni Pone. He worked for the government so many people knew him….and so I added Pone at the end of my name so we can have the same surname. And I have used both names ever since.

The early years

I was vaccinated against typhoid, small box and a few others, I cannot remember, when I was in Primary School. I was less than 10 years old at the time. I distinctly remember being told, by the nurses who did the vaccination, that I may experience some discomfort and even a fever after the vaccination but I will recover fully. It did happen, I noticed having a temperature in the evening of the same day but it was gone by morning.

Education and Career

After high school, I moved to Auckland, New Zealand to continue my studies at the Mt Albert Grammar School and the University of Auckland, graduating in May, 1985 with a Bachelor of Science. I returned to Tonga and started working for the Ministry of Agriculture, Fisheries and Forests (MAFF), in June 1985, as an

Agriculture Officer/Plant Pathologist. In 1986, the disease problems of vanilla was becoming a problem in Tonga, so I returned to Auckland University to do my research there. The project also included a Master of Science degree upon presentation of the results. My programme was eligible for an Honors classification so it was a very good result. My work on vanilla, kava and squash viruses, during the subsequent years, was recognized by the MAFF, and Tongan Government, with a promotion to the post of Senior Plant Virologist in 1991. The results are published in **Scientific Journals** and my book called **Plant Protection in the Pacific** books 1 & 2, both books are available from amazon.com

In March 1992, I was appointed to the position of Fellow in Tissue Culture at the University of the South Pacific (USP), European Union (EU) funded Pacific Regional Agriculture Project (PRAP) 7, Alafua, Apia, Samoa . The project collected popular Pacific crops for storage *in vitro,* and research, to help USP member countries during disaster management programmes such as hurricane recovery. My job was to maintain *in vitro* collections like the sweet potato/kumara (*Ipomea batatas*), bananas (*Musa sp*), vanilla (*Vanilla fragrans*), yams (*Dioscorea alata, Dioscorea esculenta*) and my colleagues would look after the taro (*Colocasia esculenta*), cassava (*Manihot esculenta*) and other germplasm.

I was also responsible for sending tissue culture plantlets to USP member countries upon request. The Senior Fellow, Dr Mary Taylor (United Kingdom) made working very easy, as everything has been organized and provided.

During my 'spare time', I also managed to carry out some research. The results are published in my third book called **Plant Protection in the Pacific 3**, tissue culture. This book is also available, in print, from amazon.com.

I joined the South Pacific Commission (SPC) Plant Protection Service, in April 1993, as its Plant Protection Advisor and Head/Co-ordinator. I was responsible, as co-ordinator, for many multi-million dollar projects including the **$NZ 5 million SPC/EU Pacific Plant Protection Project as its Manager.**

Its activities/role included;
1. Tissue Culture
2. Biological Control (in collaboration with the SPC/German Biological Control Project)
3. Biosecurity Training
4. Plant Protection Training
5. Provision of Plant Protection equipment and computers to member countries
6. Plant Protection Information dissemination/Library/Publications
7. Satellite communications with NPPOs/staff
8. Administration/management

9. Liaison with National Plant Protection Organizations (NPPO) and Regional Plant Protection Organizations (RPPO)

10. Advise the SPC Management on Plant Protection Issues of Concern

11. Organize regional/international meetings of subject matter specialists and experts on Plant Protection (We had a total of 11 meetings/seminars/workshops with up to 70 expert participants from around the world).

I was also appointed to the Panel of Experts on Biosecurity at the Food and Agriculture Organization (FAO), Rome, United Nations; for a total of about 7 years even though I 'left' (due to the vaccine injury), before my term was completed. I was also the representative of the Pacific Plant Protection Organization at the Technical Consultations of the Regional Plant Protection Organizations which meet every two years at FAO, United Nations, Rome.

The other projects included;

1. The FAO/SPC Regional Fruit Fly Project based in Fiji, managed by Mr Allan Allwood (Australia) (budget $US1 million)

Fruit flies are major pest problems in many Pacific Islands restricting the export of many produce and fruits. This project researched various ways to overcome the fruit fly problem.

2. SPC/EU Taro Beetle Project based in the Solomon Islands, managed by Dr Brian Thistleton (United Kingdom) (budget $SI 1.5 million)

Taro beetle is a major problem in many Melanesian countries including Papua New Guinea, Solomon Islands, Vanuatu and Fiji. The project did research on ways to control the taro beetle including chemicals and biological means.

3. SPC/German Regional Biological Control Project based in Fiji, managed by

Dr Jurgen Schaeffer (Germany) (budget $1-5 million)

This project carried out research and training on the use of biological control and minimizing chemical use in agricultural gardens around the Pacific, especially Integrated Pest Management (IPM).

4. SPC/AUSAID Plant Protection in Micronesia Project based in Pohnpei, Federated States of Micronesia, managed by Mr Dennis Kelly (Australia) (budget $AUD700,000)

Dennis worked together with the staff of the 3 countries (Palau, Marshalls, FSM) to improve Plant Quarantine and International movements of plant products especially in and out of the Northern Pacific.

There were also other projects I added while I was Head/Coordinator. They were;

1. SPC/CAB PACINET Biosystematics Project managed by myself and Professor Tecwyn Jones of the Commonwealth Agriculture Bureau, United Kingdom. (Budget $US 8.5 million). This project was approved after I 'left' SPC, due to vaccine injury.

2. Pacific Plant Protection Organization (PPPO). I was the Acting Chief Executive of this organization, after it was approved by the 34th South Pacific Conference in 1984. Its first meeting was held at the Tanoa Hotel, Nadi, Fiji in February 1996. (budget by SPC Secretariat)

3. The SPC/ACIAR Taro Leaf Blight Project managed by myself and Dr Paul Ferrar of the Australian Centre for International Agriculture Research. (budget $AUD 1 million). I recommended to Dr Paul Ferrar, Co-ordinator of ACIAR that this project should be done in Samoa just before I left SPC in 1996.

Reasons for 'leaving SPC'.

After the problems began with the first vaccination in about April/May 1996, I consider myself 'migrated' with my family to New Zealand in June, 1996 at the end of my first contract. I wanted to stay in Auckland and sort out my health.

All the positions on core budget, which included my job as the Plant Protection Advisor, had been advertised in a 'restructuring exercise'. I advised the Secretariat General of my intention to stay in New Zealand but I did not advise him of my health problem....because the Doctor had told me after the tests that there is nothing wrong with me.

Purpose

The purpose of this background is to impress upon the reader that this is not a fanciful claim or the ravings of a maniac. This is an account of a highly successful scientist who understands the implications for the Health Industry, and the public, of what I am saying in this book.

THE 27 MEMBER COUNTRIES OF THE SOUTH PACIFIC COMMISSION.

During my time at the South Pacific Commission the member countries were; 1. American Samoa 2. Australia 3. Cook Islands 4. Federated States of Micronesia 5. Fiji 6. France 7.French Polynesia 8. Guam 9. Kiribati 10. Marshall Is. 11. Nauru 12. New Caledonia 13. New Zealand 14. Papua New Guinea 15. Niue 16. Northern Marianas 17. Palau 18. Pitcairn Is.19. Samoa 20. Solomon Islands 21. Tonga 22. Tokelau 23.Tuvalu 24. United Kingdom 25. United States of America 26. Vanuatu 27. Wallis and Futuna

All the countries are represented at the South Pacific Conference, which met once every two years. It is where all the important decisions are made.

CHAPTER 2. Vaccines and how they work and the problems they cause.

A vaccine is described in the online encyclopedia* as;

A vaccine is a biological preparation that provides active acquired immunity to a particular disease. A vaccine typically contains an agent that resembles a disease-causing microorganism and is often made from weakened or killed forms of the microbe, its toxins, or one of its surface proteins. The agent stimulates the body's immune system to recognize the agent as a threat, destroy it, and to further recognize and destroy any of the microorganisms associated with that agent that it may encounter in the future. Vaccines can be prophylactic (example: to prevent or ameliorate the effects of a future infection by a natural or "wild" pathogen), or therapeutic (e.g., vaccines against cancer).

The administration of vaccines is called vaccination. Vaccination is the most effective method of preventing infectious diseases; widespread immunity due to vaccination is largely responsible for the worldwide eradication of smallpox and the restriction of diseases such as polio, measles and tetanus from much of the world. The effectiveness of vaccination has been widely studied and verified; for example, the influenza vaccine, the HPV vacccine and the chicken pox vaccine. The World Health Organization (WHO) reports that licensed vaccines are currently available for twenty-five different reventable vaccines.

Although vaccines has been touted to be the savior of human kind, there is an increasing number of people who claim otherwise, for very good reasons.

The following two articles by 'Sarah' and from the 'online educational page' of the Philadelphia College of Physicians are examples of the thousands of material available on the pros and cons of vaccination. The articles have been edited and amended by the author to suit this publication but the essential and important contents were untouched.

The addition of these 'free online articles' to this book is necessary to add the importance…and urgency… of why we should take action on this issue of vaccine injury.

The second article also include compensation programmes in the United States in cases where the cause of the 'serious side effects' or 'deaths' was determined to be due to the vaccine.

ARTICLE NUMBER 1.

THE HEALTHY HOME ECONOMIST
an 'online page by Sarah'.

Six reasons not to vaccinate;

Vaccination is an extremely controversial topic these days. Whatever side of the aisle you may fall with regard to your opinion about vaccination, one thing is for certain. The choice to vaccinate or not vaccinate is a decision that has the potential to greatly impact the health of you and most importantly, your children for the rest of their lives.
As a result, this decision should not be taken lightly and it should not be made in a vacuum. In other words, don't just take your pediatrician's word that shots are safe. It is possible for doctors to be wrong. They are human, after all. In reality, your doctor is simply parroting the standard line about vaccination from the American Medical Association (AMA) playbook. If you think you are getting their honest assessment, think again.
You should neither assume shots are dangerous just because your friend down the street doesn't vaccinate her kids.
The key here is education; making an informed decision by investigating the facts with an open mind and knowing exactly what you are getting yourself into before you commit to do anything.
With that in mind, the list below will briefly detail to you the reasons why I did not vaccinate my own children and will never consider a shot for them for any reason even in the event of a so called "pandemic." Please remember that I come from a medical family. My own Father (retired) is a MD as is my brother and my cousin (who was a pediatrician, now deceased). My husband's mother is a

nurse. There is no shortage of opinions on this subject in my family, I can assure you.

So, don't use family pressure as an excuse to do what you need to do once you investigate the facts for yourself and make an informed decision. There is no more foolish choice than to do something because it is someone else's wishes and not your own.   It is your body, after all and these are your children. There is no one on earth who knows what is best for them except you and your spouse – not even and most especially not your doctor! Make your decisions feeling confident in this knowledge.

Reason Number 1. Pharmaceutical Companies Can't Be Trusted (Ever)

Let's just list a couple of the (many) times over the past 10 years where a drug or drug regimen has been deemed unsafe and downright dangerous and yet the pharmaceutical companies covered it up FOR YEARS in order to continue raking in the profits for as long as possible.   This should be an easy task.

How about hormone replacement therapy for women?   The standard of care for a menopausal woman for over 40 years was HRT.   Even women with no complaints were advised that this treatment was helpful as it reduced chances for a heart attack and cancer and even helped them feel younger.   Were any, I repeat ANY of these claims true? Not a whit. Breast cancer risk is doubled for women on HRT,   41% increased risk for stroke, 29% increased risk of heart attack, and the list goes on and on.

How about Vioxx?   Before this dangerous drug that caused thousands of deaths from heart attack and stroke was finally removed from the market, evidence surfaced that Merck had withheld information and even doctored reports on its dangers years before. As of November 2007, Merck had agreed to pay $4.85 billion to settle approximately 27,000 cases from victims claiming injury or death of a family member using Vioxx. While this is a huge sum of money, in reality it represents less than one year's profits for Merck. Does it pay for a drug company to lie about a drug's safety and efficacy? You betcha. The risk of payouts to victims from getting sued is lower than the lure of huge and long lasting profits while a drug's patent protection remains in effect.

Reason Number 2. ALL Vaccines are Loaded with Chemicals and Heavy Metals

Here is a list of the damaging ingredients in vaccines on the market today verified either by independent testing and/or listed on vaccine inserts:
Nagalase, squalene, polysorbate 80, glyphosate (Roundup), e-coli, MSG, antifreeze, phenol (used as a disinfectant), formaldehyde (cancer causing and used to embalm), aluminum (associated with alzheimer's disease and seizures), glycerin (toxic to the kidney, liver, can cause lung damage, gastrointestinal damage and death), lead, cadmium, sulfates, yeast proteins, antibiotics, acetone (used in nail polish
remover), neomycin and streptomycin. And the ingredient making the press is thimerosol (more toxic than mercury, a preservative still used in many vaccines, not easily eliminated, can cause severe neurological damage as well as other life threatening autoimmune disease). These vaccines are grown and strained through animal or human tissue, like monkey and dog kidney tissue, chick embryo, calf serum, human diploid cells (the dissected organs of forcibly aborted fetuses), pig blood, horse blood and rabbit brain.

Reason Number 3. Vaccinated Children are the Unhealthiest, Most Chronically Sick Children

A comprehensive survey of nearly 12,000 children in the USA and Europe was conducted in 2010. The research revealed the truth about the health of vaccinated vs unvaccinated kids. The conclusion? Vaccinated children are more chronically ill than unvaccinated children with rates for autism, ear infections, ADHD, asthma and allergies as much as 30% higher than unvaxed children.

Reason Number 4. Other Countries Are Waking Up to the Dangers of Vaccination

In 1975, Japan raised its minimum vax age to 2 years old. The country's infant mortality subsequently plummeted to such low levels that Japan now enjoys one of the lowest level in the Western world (#3 at last look). In comparison, the United States' infant mortality rate is #33.

In Australia, the flu vaccine was suspended in April 2010 for children under 5 because an alarming number of children were showing up in the emergency rooms with febrile convulsions or other vaccine reactions within hours of getting this shot.

In the UK, they don't even require the chicken pox vaccine because it causes so many health problems not just for children, but also triggers the grave risk of a shingles epidemic for adults. By the way, the shingles vaccine doesn't even work, which is likely why the UK continues to not offer the varicella vaccine to children.

Reason Number 5. Numerous Vaccines Have Already Had Problems/Been Removed from the Market

Here is a brief list of some of the vaccines that have caused serious injury in recent years.

In Feb 2002, GlaxoSmithKline removed the (1) Lyme Disease vaccine from the market citing poor sales when in fact a number of people who received the vaccine reported symptoms worse than the disease itself such as incurable arthritis or neurological impairment.

(2) The Rotavirus vaccine (Rotashield) was removed from the market in 1999 due to an association between the vaccine and life threatening bowel obstruction or twisting of the bowl! Interestingly, my pediatrician at the time (who was a lifelong friend of our family) had highly recommended that this vaccine be given to my newborn baby at the time.   I trusted my instincts and said no to the shot – am I glad I did! My pediatrician (remember, lifelong family friend) subsequently dropped me as a patient. Guess he wasn't such a friend after all! This article contains the full story about pediatricians dropping unvaccinated patients and what to do about it. Don't be bullied parents!

(3) A warning was issued concerning the second Rotavirus vaccine (Rotateq) in 2007 as it caused the same twisting of the bowel problem in 28 infants (16 of which required intestinal surgery). This second vaccine has not yet been removed from the market as far as I know.

(4) Another vaccine that has had a lot of problems but is not yet withdrawn is the Gardasil vaccine for adolescent girls. A few years ago, Merck, the 50 billion dollar pharmaceutical company and vaccine manufacturer, recalled 743,000 contaminated Gardasil shots that contained glass particles. Fainting, paralysis, slurred speech are just a few of the reactions reported and yet this vaccine continues to stay on the market. At least 1600 adverse events have been reported since its approval in 2006, yet doctors are continuing to recommend this shot to their patients. Why this vaccine hasn't already been removed from the market is astonishing. In Japan unlike the US, citizens are permitted to sue vaccine manufacturers for damages, and as of this writing, a class action lawsuit is pending against the makers of HPV vaccines.

Reason Number 6. You Can Always Get Vaccinated, But You Can Never Undo a Vaccination

Procrastination is usually considered a character flaw, but in the case of vaccination, delaying the decision for as long as possible plays to your advantage.   The longer you wait to vaccinate your child, the better.   A child's immune system continues to develop for years after birth.   The blood/brain barrier does not fully develop until adolescence.   The longer you wait, the more likely your child's immune system will be able to handle the onslaught with minimal damage.

If you don't know what to do, don't do anything! Conversely, you can never undo a vaccination. There are holistic therapies that can detox a child from the vaccine's poison, but the damage that is done can never be 100% repaired. And, I have NEVER met a fully vaccinated child that is healthier and more robust than a well nourished, unvaccinated child. Period.

While I would like to convince you to never vaccinate your child, if I can simply convince you to delay it for a few years that is certainly better than vaccinating a baby. If you can simply commit to waiting until your child is school age to vaccinate, so much the better than if you vaccinate as a toddler and so on. Time is on your side and waiting is the best policy when it comes to shots. Another vaccine alternative to consider is homeoprophylaxis. This nontoxic method to boost immunity safely is gaining rapid popularity due to the numerous scientific studies involving millions of people to support its efficacy. And, if your child starts to regress after shots, be sure to do the emergency vaccine detox recommended by developmental pediatrician Dr. Mary Megson.

By the time your child is older, more research will have been done, you will have an opportunity to learn more and become more comfortable with your decision to

wait. Who knows? Your attitude of wait and see may turn out to be permanent like mine was 20 years ago.
Books by Medical Doctors Warning Against Vaccines
It's not just well researched parents that are rebelling against vaccines, medical doctors are too!

Authored by Sarah, The Healthy Home Economist

ARTICLE NUMBER 2

This is an example of articles that are available from the Scientific Community on the subject;

An article from the College of Physicians of Philadelphia 'educational online page'.

Vaccine Side Effects and Adverse Events

1. A vaccine is a medical product. Vaccines, though they are designed to protect from disease, can cause side effects, just as any medication can.
2. Most side effects from vaccination are mild, such as soreness, swelling, or redness at the injection site. Some vaccines are associated with fever, rash, and achiness. Serious side effects are rare, but may include **seizure or life-threatening allergic reaction.**
3. A possible side effect resulting from a vaccination is known as an adverse event.
4. Each year, American babies (1 year old and younger) receive more than 10 million vaccinations. During the first year of life, a significant number of babies suffer serious, life-threatening illnesses and medical events, such as Sudden Infant Death Syndrome (SIDS). Additionally, it is during the first year that congenital conditions may become evident. Therefore, due to chance alone, many babies will experience a medical event in close proximity

to a vaccination. This does not mean, though, that the event is in fact related to the immunization. The challenge is to determine when a medical event is directly related to a vaccination.

5. The Food and Drug and Administration (FDA) and the Centers for Disease Control and Prevention (CDC) have set up systems to monitor and analyze reported adverse events and to determine whether they are likely related to vaccination.

Types of Side Effects

1. To understand the range of possible vaccination side effects events, it is useful to compare a vaccine with relatively few associated side effects, such as the vaccine for *Haemophilus* influenza type B, with a vaccine known to have many potential side effects, such as the infrequently used smallpox vaccine (given to military personnel and others who might be first responders in the event of a bioterror attack).

2. *Haemophilus* influenza type B is a bacterium that can cause serious infections, including meningitis, pneumonia, epiglottitis, and sepsis. The CDC recommends that children receive a series of Hib vaccinations starting when they are two months old.

3. Smallpox is a serious infection, fatal In 30% to 40% of cases, and caused by the Variola major or Variola minor virus. No wild smallpox cases have been reported since the 1970s. The World Health Organization has declared it eradicated.

The information below about side effects of Hib and smallpox vaccination is from the Centers for Disease Control and Prevention.

Hib Vaccine Side Effects

1. Redness, warmth, or swelling where the shot was given (up to 1 out of 4 children)
2. Fever over 101°F (up to 1 out of 20 children)
3. No serious side effects have been related to the Hib vaccine.
4. Smallpox (Vaccinia) Vaccine Side Effects
5. Mild to Moderate Problems
6. Mild rash, lasting 2-4 days.
7. Swelling and tenderness of lymph nodes, lasting 2-4 weeks after the blister has healed.
8. Fever of over 100°F (about 70% of children, 17% of adults) or over 102°F (about 15%-20% of children, under 2% of adults).
9. Secondary blister elsewhere on the body (about 1 per 1,900).

Moderate to Severe Problems

1. Serious eye infection, or loss of vision, due to spread of vaccine virus to the eye.
2. Rash on entire body (as many as 1 per 4,000).
3. Severe rash on people with eczema (as many as 1 per 26,000).
4. Encephalitis (severe brain reaction), which can lead to permanent brain damage (as many as 1 per 83,000).
5. Severe infection beginning at the vaccination site (as many as 1 per 667,000, mostly in people with weakened immune systems).
6. Death (1-2 per million, mostly in people with weakened immune systems).

For every million people vaccinated for smallpox, between 14 and 52 could have a life-threatening reaction to smallpox vaccine.

Question. How Do I Find Out the Side Effects for Different Vaccines?

Answer. When you or a child gets a vaccine, the health care provider gives you a handout known as the Vaccine Information Statement (VIS). The VIS describes common and rare side effects, if any are known, of the vaccine. Your health care provider will probably discuss possible side effects with you. VIS downloads are also available through the CDC's website.

Additional Information.

1. Package inserts produced by the vaccine manufacturer also provide information about adverse events. Additionally, these inserts usually show rates of adverse events in experimental and control groups during pre-market testing of the vaccine.

How Are Adverse Events Monitored?

1. VAERS (Vaccine Adverse Event Reporting System)
2. The CDC and FDA established The Vaccine Adverse Event Reporting System in 1990. The goal of VAERS, according to the CDC, is "to detect possible signals of adverse events associated with vaccines." (A signal in this case is evidence of a possible adverse event that emerges in the data collected.) About 30,000 events are reported each year to VAERS. Between 10% and 15% of these reports describe serious medical events that result in hospitalization, life-threatening illness, disability, or death.
3. VAERS is a voluntary reporting system. Anyone, such as a parent, a health care provider, or friend of the patient, who suspects an association between a vaccination and an adverse event may report that event and information about it to VAERS. The CDC then investigates the event and tries to find out whether the adverse event was in fact caused by the vaccination.
4. The CDC states that they monitor VAERS data to
    (i) Detect new, unusual, or rare vaccine adverse events
    (ii) Monitor increases in known adverse events

(iii) Identify potential patient risk factors for particular types of adverse events

(iv) Identify vaccine lots with increased numbers or types of reported adverse events

(v) Assess the safety of newly licensed vaccines

(vi) Not all adverse events reported to VAERS are in fact caused by a vaccination. The two occurrences may be related in time only. And, it is probable that not all adverse events resulting from vaccination are reported to VAERS. The CDC states that many adverse events such as swelling at the injection site are underreported. Serious adverse events, according to the CDC, "are probably more likely to be reported than minor ones, especially when they occur soon after vaccination, even if they may be coincidental and related to other causes."

VAERS has successfully identified several rare adverse events related to vaccination. Among them are;

1. An intestinal problem after the first vaccine for rotavirus was introduced (the vaccine was withdrawn in 1999)

2. Neurologic and gastrointestinal diseases related to yellow fever vaccine

Additionally, according to Plotkin *et al.*, VAERS identified a need for further investigation of MMR association with a blood clotting disorder, encephalopathy after MMR, and syncope after immunization (Plotkin S A *et al.* Vaccines, 5thed. Philadelphia: Saunders, 2008).

Vaccine Safety Datalink
The CDC established this system in 1990. The VSD is a collection of linked databases containing information from large medical groups. The linked databases allow officials to gather data about

vaccination among the populations served by the medical groups. Researchers can access the data by proposing studies to the CDC and having them approved.

The VSD has some drawbacks. For example, few completely unvaccinated children are listed in the database. The medical groups providing information to VSD may have patient populations that are not representative of large populations in general. Additionally, the data come not from randomized, controlled, blinded trials but from actual medical practice. Therefore, it may be difficult to control and evaluate the data.

Rapid Cycle Analysis;

 Is a program of the VSD, launched in 2005. It monitors real-time data to compare rates of adverse events in recently vaccinated people with rates among unvaccinated people. The system is used mainly to monitor new vaccines. Among the new vaccines being monitored in Rapid Cycle Analysis are the conjugated meningococcal vaccine, rotavirus vaccine, MMRV vaccine, Tdap vaccine, and the HPV vaccine. Possible associations between adverse events and vaccination are then studied further.

Article on compensation programmes on vaccine injury also by the College of Physicians of Philadelphia 'educational online page'.

Vaccine Injury Compensation Programs

1. The Vaccine Information Sheet for a vaccine against human papillomavirus

Centers for Disease Control and Prevention

1. No medical intervention is completely risk free. Vaccines, though they are designed to protect from disease, can cause side effects that range from mild to serious. The most common side effects from vaccination are soreness, swelling, or redness at the injection site. Some vaccines are associated with fever, rash, and achiness. Serious side effects from vaccination are rare, but may include **life-threatening allergic reaction, seizure**, and even death.

2. When vaccines first began to be widely used, people who experienced serious side effects from vaccination had little recourse to compensation from manufacturers, physicians, or the government. This was particularly a problem when vaccine production techniques were in their infancy and contamination of vaccines occasionally occurred during or after manufacture. Since the passage in 1902 of the U.S. Biologics Control Act, which initiated the regulation of vaccines, such problems with negligence in manufacture have declined greatly.

3. As product liability law evolved during the 20th century, it eventually provided an avenue for compensation for individuals harmed by vaccines: they could sue a manufacturer for harm caused by an improperly made vaccine, or they could sue a physician for administering a vaccine when it was contraindicated. In the United States, the civil court system applies the principles of tort law to these suits.

4. This rest of this article addresses programs that compensate individuals for adverse clinical events that are known to be caused by properly manufactured vaccines. Because governments have an interest in maintaining public health by means of vaccination, many, including the U.S. government, have developed no-fault systems for compensating people who have been adversely affected by certain vaccines. These people, to some degree, have

assumed the risk of adverse event on behalf of the society in which they live. Therefore, many governments have adopted the position that it is fair and reasonable to compensate those who are harmed by properly manufactured vaccines.

For example, The Cutter Incident and Resulting Lawsuits

1. Individuals harmed by properly manufactured vaccines had few options for compensation before an important court case in the 1950s addressed the issue. In 1955 about 200 people were paralyzed and ten died after contracting polio from the Salk polio vaccine, certain lots of which contained virus that had not been inactivated in spite of manufacturers' adherence to federal government standards. The event came to be known as the Cutter Incident, after the manufacturer of one of the implicated vaccines. Many injured people and their families filed lawsuits against vaccine manufacturers, and most of the cases were settled out of court with monetary awards by the manufacturers. One case, Gottsdanker v. Cutter Laboratories, was heard on appeal by the California Supreme Court, and the justices upheld a jury ruling that although Cutter Laboratories was not negligent in its design or manufacture of the vaccine, **the company was financially responsible for the harm the vaccine caused**. It was a significant ruling, and many similar awards followed in other cases. No standards existed, however, for determining when a vaccine caused a clinical event or was simply associated temporally with it—that is, whether the event happened to occur after vaccination without a causal relationship. Juries decided these matters on a case by case basis, at times with little medical or scientific support for claims of vaccine injury causation.

DPT Lawsuits

Through the 1970s and 1980s, the number of lawsuits brought against vaccine manufacturers increased dramatically, and manufacturers made large payouts to individuals and families claiming vaccine injury, particularly from the combined diphtheria-pertussis-tetanus (DPT) immunization. In this environment of increasing litigation, mounting legal fees, and large jury rewards, many pharmaceutical companies left the vaccine business. In fact, by the end of 1984, only one U.S. company still manufactured the DPT vaccine, and other vaccines were losing manufacturers as well.

NCVIA/NCVIP (National Childhood Vaccine Injury Act)

In October 1986, the U.S. Congress responded to the precarious situation in the vaccine market by passing the National Childhood Vaccine Injury Act (NCVIA). The act included a number of regulations related to informed consent and adverse event reporting. For example, the act required that providers administering certain vaccines provide a Vaccine Information Statement (VIS) to the vaccine recipient or a legal guardian. The VIS lists the risks and benefits of a particular vaccine. The NCVIA also established a system for reporting suspected vaccine-related adverse events. This system, the Vaccine Adverse Event Reporting System (VAERS), is described. Additionally, the act contained provisions for a program that would fairly and efficiently compensate individuals harmed by certain vaccines that were properly manufactured. Such a system, it was hoped, would stabilize the legal environment for manufacturers, allowing them to limit their liability, better anticipate their legal costs, and reduce potential barriers to research into new vaccines.

The U.S. Department of Health and Human Services (DHHS) established this system, the National Vaccine Injury Compensation Program (NVICP), in 1988. NVICP is funded by a tax of $0.75 per vaccine dose, collected from vaccine manufacturers by the U.S. Department of the Treasury. The NVICP does not cover all vaccines; however, vaccines routinely given to children as part of the recommended immunization schedule are included, and some adult vaccines are covered as well.

Under the NVICP, those claiming a vaccine injury from a covered vaccine cannot sue a vaccine manufacturer without first filing a claim with the U.S. Court of Federal Claims. Certain medical events are presumed to be side effects of vaccination as long as no other cause is found. The claim filer is reimbursed according to a formula, provided that all the medical records meet NCVIA standards and that review by the U.S. Department of Justice determines that all legal standards have been met. If a claim is denied, or if the claim is approved and the claimant rejects the compensation, only then may the claimant file a civil lawsuit.

The National Childhood Vaccine Injury Act Reporting and Compensation Tables (VIT) list each covered vaccine, its associated adverse events, and the allowable interval from vaccination to onset of event. The table of vaccine injuries has been formulated on the analysis of extensive data collected by the safety system, which includes reports to VAERS, prospective studies in HMOs by CDC, and studies by academic investigators. Examples of compensable injuries are intussusception within 30 days of receipt of oral, rhesus-based rotavirus vaccine, brachial neuritis within 0-28 days of receipt of tetanus toxoid containing vaccines, anaphylaxis within 0-4 hours of receipt of a variety of vaccines, and so on. The VIT is subject to review by DHHS, and vaccine injuries may be added to and removed from the tables depending on the best available evidence. Seizure disorder after DPT vaccination, which was the cause of many successful lawsuits against vaccine manufacturers before the NVICP, was removed from the list of compensable events in 1995 because of lack of evidence supporting a link. As new vaccines are added to the childhood immunization schedule, any associated adverse events are added to the VIT as well.

Compensation payments from NVICP have averaged $782,136 per successful claim through 2011, with an additional $113 million dispersed to pay attorney fees and legal costs (the act awards attorney fees and costs for unsuccessful claims provided that the litigants bring their claims in good faith and upon a reasonable basis, as well as for successful claims). Compensation for a death resulting from vaccination is capped at $250,000. As of December 1, 2011, the program had awarded $2.35 billion in 2,810 separate claims, including compensation for 390 deaths.

Autism Omnibus Proceeding

Beginning around 2001, hundreds and then thousands of families began to petition NVICP claiming that their children's autism resulted from vaccination. (See the article The History of Anti-vaccination Movements, and specifically the section "The Measles, Mumps, Rubella (MMR) Vaccine Controversy" for a discussion of the origin of these claims.) To deal with the volume of these petitions, and to address the assertion that a causal relationship existed between vaccination and autism, the NVICP established a special program in 2002 called the Omnibus Autism Proceeding, housed within the U.S. Court of Federal Claims Office of Special Masters.

The OAP consolidated many of the autism claims into three test cases that rested on different theories of causation. (i) The first test case addressed the issue of whether measles-mumps-rubella (MMR) vaccine alone or given along with thimerosal-containing vaccines (TCVs) is a causal factor in development of autism. (Thimerosal is an ethylmercury compound that was a common preservative in some killed vaccines.) (ii) The second test case examined TCVs alone. (iii) The third test case was to look solely at MMR vaccines, but the case was withdrawn after parties announced that they would rely on the findings of the first test case.

A special master issued the first opinion in the OAP on theory one in 2009. The ruling found, in three test cases consolidated into theory one, that MMR vaccine given alone or with TCVs is not a causal factor in autism. Theory two was decided in 2010, with a finding of no causal relation between TCVs and autism. Appeals by petitioners in the two test cases have been unsuccessful, and autism has not been added to the VIT for any vaccine.

Petitioners remaining in the OAP must submit new evidence or theories of causation of autism by vaccines, abide by the existing rulings as their cases are dismissed by the OAP, or exit the program to pursue other legal options. To date, no other theories of causes have been ruled upon, though petitioners are attempting to advance them.

Outside the United States

Many developed nations have instituted similar programs to the NVICP in the United States. Their means of funding varies, as do other details of the programs, such as vaccines and adverse events covered and how the programs handle petitioners' legal fees. In some cases (Germany and Switzerland) the state, rather than the national government, administers the program. And in countries with national health plans, **vaccine injury compensation** is a secondary source of support, as basic health care is provided at no or very little cost. In general, developing nations have not established compensation systems for vaccine injuries. Attention, however, is being paid to the need to monitor adverse events after immunization as GAVI, PATH, the World Health Organization, and other NGOs continue their efforts to fund and deliver vaccines to the developing world. Such efforts may eventually lead to compensation systems.

Conclusion

The vaccine market has stabilized since the passage of the NCVIA and the establishment of the NVCIP. In the United States, six manufacturers supply most of the standard childhood and adult vaccines, and a handful of smaller companies and organizations supply other, less commonly used vaccines. Occasional vaccine shortages do occur (such as with influenza vaccine in 2003 through 2005) but these shortages may be due to a combination of factors without a strong connection to liability issues, such as the effect of corporate mergers, the level of government reimbursement for vaccines in the federally funded Vaccine for Children program, and regulatory issues.

CHAPTER 3. What happened?

+ - the names of the clinic and anyone involved will be disguised for legal and privacy purposes. It is not the intention of this book to smear, degrade or destroy the reputation of the Health Staff involved.

In April 1996, I came with my family to Auckland, New Zealand on 'an end of contract leave' from my job at the South Pacific Commission, Suva Office, Fiji. I also wanted to have a health check done and was told that I need to be vaccinated against Hepatitis B because I don't have any anti-bodies present in my blood. It was a protective measure, in my view.

The vaccination plan was for the first shot in April/May, the next one in 3 months and the last in 6 months. My first vaccination was done around that time (April/May) at the Glenfield Clinic[+].

The first vaccination and dizzy spells

After the first vaccination, I noticed that I was experiencing some dizzy spells as if I am 'blacking out' while standing. I would sway to and fro and correct my balance as soon as I was awake again. I bought a Fruit and Vegetable Shop, in June/July, 1996 after deciding to stay in Auckland with my family. During the hours I spent alone in the shop, I was momentarily 'blacking out' regularly but recovered quickly before I collapse to the floor. In any one day, I counted 3 or more episodes. I decided to visit a Health Clinic in Northcote and explained to the Doctor there the dizzy spells I was experiencing and my recent Hepatitis B vaccination. He booked me into the lab next door where I had some tests done. A blood test was also done, but the Doctor could not find anything wrong with me. The final two vaccinations went ahead. I cannot remember discussing the dizzy spells with the Glenfield Clinic. I might have mentioned it.

I bought then sold a business because of my health problems

I decided to join a Health Supplement Company to sell their products and also take the supplements to try and cure my dizzy spells. I sold the fruit and vegetable shop because I was doing a lot of hard work, early hours driving to Turner's and Growers for the morning auction and so on. I was usually exhausted at the end of the day. Some of my major customers were also owing me 'big' money and I was getting really stressed. In fact, it was about $22,000 in total! That can stress any healthy person who doesn't have my dizzy spells on top of it!

I bought antioxidants, fish oil and aloe vera products and took them daily while selling them to friends and family. Over a period of about one to two years, I noticed that the dizzy spells have disappeared. I stopped selling the Health Supplements and decided to get a 'job'.

My first trip overseas after migrating to New Zealand in 1996

I visited my family in Fiji and Tonga, for the first time in 6 years, in 2002 and 2003. Being an agriculture person, I like going to the family farm allotment to do some work there.

The first symptom of allergy to coconut water

One day, on my return in the afternoon, probably about 3 o'clock, I almost completely lost control of my motor movements. About one kilometre from home I could not feel my hands and arms and I could barely move them. I almost crashed the ute. When I got home, I was in shock, I got out of the ute but moved like a disabled person who cannot control his legs and body. I tried really hard to move 10 metres, finally collapsing on a concrete slab outside my parent's house and lie there for about one to two hours. It rained for an hour or so but I could not move. Finally, after about one to two hours I could feel that I can get up and go inside to have a shower. That event was completely unexpected, I have never lost control of my body movements before. I did not tell anybody about it, and decided to return to Auckland.

Some months later, I was again back at Northshore hospital, Auckland, for pain problems with my feet. They did the usual blood tests, and while lying on the bed, the nurse came and told me something that really blew me away. I was allergic to coconut water! I remember that day where I 'lost feeling' in my legs and arms, I had drunk a lot of coconut water, probably up to 10 green coconuts the whole day!. It was a very hot day and I was very sweaty planting some taro and cassava. I have been drinking coconuts for years as a child and this news that I am allergic to it was a huge shock.

Swollen elbows and ankles

I noticed some pain on top of my right foot, then both my ankles and elbows became swollen but I could not feel any pain. After about a month or two the swelling subsided. That happened quite regularly. Then one morning I woke up with my foot 'on fire', I have never felt such intense pain before. I went to Northshore Hospital and got an injection done on my foot and the pain disappeared! My health deteriorated quickly. First, I was getting regular pain in the feet and ankles, I was also feeling 'down' many times a day.

Visiting my parents

I had visited Tonga 4 times between August, 2011 and 25 February, 2015. During those visits I would always come back barely alive. It started with sore ankles and knees and then my whole health just deteriorated to the point where I thought I might die. My only saving point was the knowledge I learned during my days as a Health Product salesperson. I learned some really important knowledge about supplements and what kind of food have high anti-oxidants and nutrients that can improve my health. Looking back on those days now, I think the nurse had a good point, I was allergic to coconut water….and probably other

Tongan foods. The hot weather did not help.

My father and mother's deaths

These 'personal health' episodes took place between 1996, after my vaccine injection and 2005, a period of 9-10 years. The news of my father's death in 2005 came at a time when I was 'completely lost' in the health problem. I could not fly to Tonga to attend his funeral because I just felt I will not be able to manage my own health while I was there. I felt my body was a complete wreck with painful knees, ankles and even fingers and fists. My terrible feelings of being 'depressed' did not help. My physical condition was just very bad at the time.
However, I was able to attend my Mum's funeral in 2012 and although I was financially unable to help, I provided much needed moral support to my siblings.

Trying to be healthier

I started exercising, by walking on the road every week and felt a bit better. I walked at least once a week for up to 3 hours at a time. I read Nelson Mandela's biography and he was walking 4 hours every morning before work. He was the President of South Africa and 70 years old!. That book was a huge inspiration to me. I thought of Mandela's 'can do' attitude and his 27 years in jail….my problem seem insignificant.

Information collection trip

During my 2015 visit (January - February) to collect information for my books, I also fell very ill after 2 weeks. I had swollen and sore ankles, sore knees and elbows. I was in bed for about 2 weeks. Fortunately, I lived with my aunt and relatives who helped me. My normal medication I brought from New Zealand had run out. I used local medicine from the hospital, and panadol from the local shops, which allowed me to return to

Auckland, more or less in good health but I felt like I just came back from the dead.

My thighs were on fire!

I also remember sometime after that I was lying in my room screaming because both my thighs were just 'on fire', the pain was so intense that I cried out every time it happens. I got my wife to buy some Voltaren from the Pharmacy which helped relieve it. I have never had this problem before or since.

Gout

From 2016-2018, I rarely have gout attacks. The Doctor had told me it is gout. I got some medicine from the Doctor which helped a lot and I was symptom free for months!

I ran out of medicine

While writing this book, I have a swollen right ankle and I can barely walk. My medicine from the Doctor (sodium dichlofinac) had finished 3 months ago, and I am still waiting for a repeat. I made a request to the receptionist but they have not called me back. We have moved out of Northcote to a new house in Bayview and that might be the reason. I called them again but they seem to be angry with me at the moment.

Dieting and Supermarket Medicine

I am just using a diet regiment and supermarket medicine (panadol and nuromol) which worked for a while until I decided to break with my diet tradition and the gout came back! I bought some supplements and will try to use natural methods to improve the supermarket medicine effectiveness. I had bought a bottle of tart cherry capsules and I think it is working. The swelling on my right angle, which was 3 times bigger than my left ankle, has gone down after taking just 2 capsules of freeze dried tart cherry the previous evening.

I don't want to go back to the Doctor (at our old clinic in Northcote) who did not give me any prescriptions during my last 2 visits. I might even join a new clinic. I think maybe he wants me to slow down on the pills, which I think can be dangerous if I take too many of them. I am trying to reduce my dependence on the medicine.

Requests for help from the SPC was declined

I had made a request to my last employer, the South Pacific Commission, now known as the Secretariat for the Pacific Community, for help. I wrote to the Secretary General sometime between 2,000 and 2006 and the Human Resource Manager called me back and explained that they cannot help. Even though I received the first vaccination during my last 2 months, in April/May, as a staff member of the South Pacific Commission, the HRM said they cannot help.

Request for help from the Tongan Government was declined

I also wrote to the Prime Minister of Tonga, Prince 'Ulkalala, Lavaka, 'Ata for some help. I received a letter back from the PM's Office for more information and I sent them some printouts of an article about 'vaccine injury'. I never heard back from them again. The Prince resigned as Prime Minister in February, 2006 and I did not follow up with the new PM, Dr Fred Sevele. I thought that he might do something about it since he was a former SPC staff member…but nothing happened.

The New Zealand Situation

The New Zealand Government does provide many relief assistance to unemployed and sick residents and citizens. These include an unemployment benefit, sickness benefit, reduced medical costs, much free medical care…so I was lucky in a way because I received a lot of assistance locally in Auckland.

The issue should have been raised at the South Pacific Conference

 I thought that Tonga should have raised the issue at the South Pacific Conference because it is very important that this kind of health problem…and issue… does not arise again in the future to SPC staff members. Their families who are affected financially by it, deserve better. I was insured in the SPC Staff insurance programme. There are also other areas that could have been explored such as what happens to SPC staff members whose health and career are destroyed by such unexpected medical misadventure. As I have pointed out with the articles in Chapter 2, there are programmes in the United States, for example, that can be used by the SPC to compensate staff members whose lives and career are destroyed and also help their families financially. **All they have to do is pass a 'resolution' in the South Pacific Conference that they will help such staff members and adopt the USA**

policy on compensating them. It is that easy.

The problem is finding a SP Conference member/representative who is convinced and willing to fight for such a cause and persuade the Conference to approve such a resolution. I thought the Secretary General should have acted on receiving my letter and do something about it 10-20 years ago.

CHAPTER 4. The symptoms

The symptoms that I have mentioned already are all described in the articles on vaccine injury, in Chapter 2. They do not occur normally on their own. They include;

1. Dizzy spells and momentary 'blackouts'
2. Swollen ankles and elbows with no pain
3. Tiredness and achiness. I get really tired with an aching back after sitting on the computer for 30 minutes or more.
4. Loss of feeling in arms and legs that last about 30 minutes to one hour (i.e. loss of motor movements).
5. Skin lesions that appear like 'tinea' but are 'raised' above the skin surface, almost like a rash
6. Gout like symptoms that eventually became full blown gout with pain in the joints

7. Other painful symptoms on my back, thighs, hands and stomach that are not consistent with gout symptoms
8. Intense pain on feet and thighs
9. Fungal growth on both big toe nails (this may be due to less immune response because I have never had this problem before the vaccination)
10. Forgetfulness (I noticed this as a kind of surprise because I have a very good photographic memory, but it just appears out of nowhere)
11. Loss of 'motor' movement or control of limbs. For example, I play the ukulele and guitar and I have noticed that sometimes my motor movements are 'clumsy'. That is, I don't play as well as I normally do.
12. I am also 'rapidly' losing my ability to read without glasses. I normally read without glasses.
13. Allergic reaction to coconut water and other foods (I sometimes feel really sick and sleepy after eating)

CHAPTER 5. Twenty years of suffering

From April 1996 to to-day, 25 July 2018, it has been over 20 years. During that time, I have lost my good health and my ability to earn money to look after my family. My income during that time is probably less than $NZ10,000 per year, average. When I was at the South Pacific Commission (SPC), as a Professional Grade I staff, I was earning about $US66,000 per year, as its Plant Protection Advisor and Co-ordinator of the Plant Protection Service.

Fortunately, for my family, my wife works and earn enough to get us food on the table and a roof over our heads. All the bills have to be juggled but there are plenty of letters from the debt collectors, sometimes. I try to run a small business doing lawns and small contracts to make some extra money to help.

I now have 3 children, there were only 2 young ones at SPC, and 6 grand-children.

I write books most of the time to occupy and keep my mind sharp as well as build up a passive income. I know it is good for me because there is such a huge difference, in terms of overall quality, between my first book and my current publications. I am really surprised. I have improved a lot....mentally and physically.

Although we are always short of money, as a family, we are much happier now than before. Things are looking good for the family's future. The business environment is getting better.

CHAPTER 6. What shall we do about it?

The United States programme for compensating vaccine injury, as outlined by the article from the Philadelphia School of Physicians, in Chapter 2, should be adopted by the Secretariat for the Pacific Community (SPC) for future interventions in the event that a staff member is affected. There may be areas that need improvement or changed but the idea is good.

The United States of America and the donor country members of the SPC should put up a fund for helping staff members with such problems in the future.

As you can see from my story in Chapter 1, the SPC staff members do a lot of good work for the Pacific region and its peoples and deserve to be treated with respect and kindness. In my case, I was handling a huge workload but I really enjoyed it.

As you have seen from my case, it is a long and lifetime of health problems. It is not right to say, that my health problems are not due to the vaccine, that I am just unhealthy because I was very healthy, all my life, before the vaccine injury. It is also not right to say that nothing will happen in the future because it will. Just read the cases that are now filling up cyberspace.

What the SPC Conference should be saying, is 'we should have been doing this in the 1950s when the first cases of vaccine injury and death occurred' in the United States. It has been 60 years in the making but it will finally be done. The members of the South Pacific Conference, which is the governing body of the SPC should never let this go without some action done.

The Secretariat for the Pacific Community should act 'as a matter of urgency' because it will take years for the action to be felt at the grassroots level around the Pacific. The death of two babies in Samoa, just this month (July 2018), after they have been vaccinated should put more weight to my recommendation.

CHAPTER 7 Unemployment and Financial Hardship

I thought the story would not be complete without a discussion of the unemployment and financial situation. This is the most important issue from the family and relative's point of view.

I don't want to blame anyone or sound like I blame the system or others for my problems, but I feel that this issue of unemployment and financial hardship, in our case, can be linked directly to the 'vaccine injury'.

Deciding to stay in Auckland

When it was clear to me that I have a health issue after the vaccination, I had to think of the options available to me. I was not sure that SPC will give me my job back. All the core budget jobs have been advertised. I was in the panel that selected our Agriculture Programme Manager, before I left for New Zealand, and I supported the incumbent to have another term. He would get 9 years in total. I was not sure who the panel will select in my case.

I was also not sure how serious my health problem is, I might return to Fiji and have a huge health problem there and I will not get the same kind of medical care as in New Zealand. My two young children, who were 8 and 5 years, also need some quality schooling and care. If something happens to me it would be better for my wife and kids in New Zealand because there were many government assistance programmes for families and unemployed people. There are none in Fiji.

I decided to inform the SG of my decision to stay in Auckland, but I did not tell him about my health issue. That was around April/May 1996. I was not sure at all what it was. The Doctor had already told me they cannot find any problems when I reported the 'dizzy spells', after the first vaccination.

Looking for a job

I checked the newspapers every week, but most jobs would not suit me. There were always many laboring jobs available but not in my specialist field. I called all the Science Departments and Companies I knew, but there were no vacancies.

I did get one interview for a Co-ordinator of Pacific Island Affairs or something like that. I was shocked at the number of interviewers there. There must have been 10 of them. What made it worse for me was, a staff member of that Ministry told me they will give the job to a current staff member. I should have walked out of there. The interview was a disaster! I was both annoyed and embarrassed that they already intend to give the job to somebody else.

I also applied to many other jobs.

I saw an article in the Northshore times that another immigrant, a woman, had applied for more than 100 jobs but was still unsuccessful!

It gives you an idea of what job seeking was like in Auckland in 1996.

Deciding to start a business

I was looking through the newspapers at the properties for sale. Some were very cheap. They were just $10-20,000 or thereabouts. I was thinking of buying 2 or 3 in the South Island and rent them out. Then I got scared that they won't find any tenants. There were just too many negative stories about empty rental houses, in the South Island, at the time.

I also checked the local Auckland properties. I liked one in South Auckland but upon visiting and viewing it, I changed my mind. Now, I feel that I should have bought them because they would be worth, at least, 20 times more.

So the only option available to me was to use our savings to start a business. I bought a cheap Fruit and Vege Shop in Royal Oak, Auckland, which was losing money, but I had an idea to import rootcrops from the islands and sell them there. I also bought the couple's truck. They got $25,000 in one week! I think they probably thought I was an angel. They were losing a lot of money and I came along and saved them!

My first container of cassava from Fiji arrived soon after. I had arranged with a friend in Fiji to supply my shop. I was the only supplier of Fijian cassava in Auckland at the time. It was a gold mine! I sold the first container in a month! Then I ordered another one.

The shop turnover, when I took over, was about $1,000 a week, barely enough to buy the stock and pay for the rent and outgoings. After a month, my turnover was $3-4,000 a week. I was making some profit from the cassava.

Then two businesses ordered 2 containers of coconuts (about 60,000 nuts) and a container of cassava and refused to pay. They owe me $22,000 and my business was suffering from the 'loss of cash'.

I had paid my father in Tonga for the two containers of coconuts at 10 cents each. He was buying them at 5 cents per nut from the growers. I pay for the freight and costs in Auckland and I sold the containers of coconuts at about 30 cents a nut. The guy got a good deal. I was selling the nuts at $1.40 in my shop! So it was a cheap deal, but he could not pay. There were always issues with his cash flow and other excuses. I had visited his factory and I thought that his concentrated coconut cream would make a killing in the local market!

It would have been a good profitable arrangement. Needless to say, we had a court case and spent all our money on the legal proceedings that we both canceled it.

Indonesia is now supplying the concentrated coconut cream in Auckland with a huge monopoly…and everyone is buying their cream! They must be laughing all the way to the bank.

I did find out, later, that the coconut processing factory owner did have two properties, but I also know that he was up to his neck in debts. He had lost his factory in the court case and I did not want to put his family out on the streets.

The guy who ordered the container of cassava was supplying Tongan cassava and he could not pay for some 'funny' reasons. I gave him my list of suppliers in Fiji, when I finally decided to close my shop.

I hear his business was saved by my 'free container' of cassava.

The same goes for the fruit shop owner and coconut factory owner's houses. I guess I was good for them but it didn't do me any good.

Job Seeking

It was back to job seeking again. I did find a lot of laboring jobs but did not get any in my field of Plant Pathology/Virology or even administration.

I could have gone back to University and 'retrained' like so many people but I guess I just had too many 'bad luck' stories. I was thinking it would not make any difference at all.

We survived with very little money over the last 20 years. My wife's parents and our relatives also helped.

I decided to become a writer. At least, I can do something I like….then also started a small lawn and garden business which is growing quickly.

I do look back and count my blessings. Nelson Mandela's story is an inspiration to me. It makes me feel I want to do something….to make a difference.

ABBREVIATIONS

1. AUSAID - Australian Agency for International Development
2. EU - European Union
3. FAO - Food and Agriculture Organization of the United Nations
4. NPPO - National Plant Protection Organizations
5. PPPO - Pacific Plant Protection Organization
6. RPPO - Regional Plant Protection Organizations
7. SG - Secretary General
8. SPC - South Pacific Commission

PICTURES OF SWOLLEN HANDS AND FEET

Although I did not intend to take pictures for this book, I do have some pictures of some symptoms.

Figure 1. A picture of my swollen left hand taken on February 2018. The swelling of my hands, elbows and ankles seem to appear at random, probably triggered by the foods I eat.

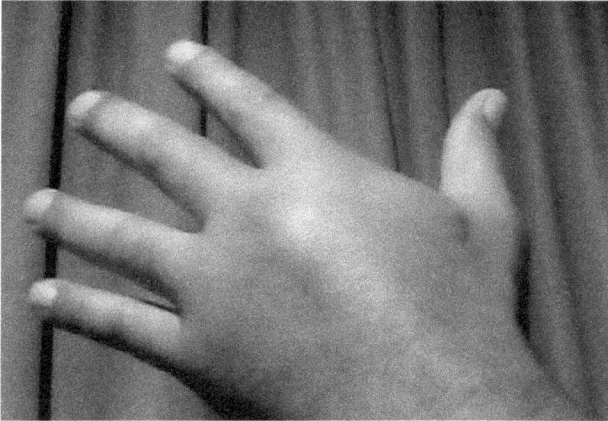

Figure 2. My swollen right foot. This picture was taken in July 2018. My ankles have been swollen 'off and on' for years. Note the swollen 2nd toe.

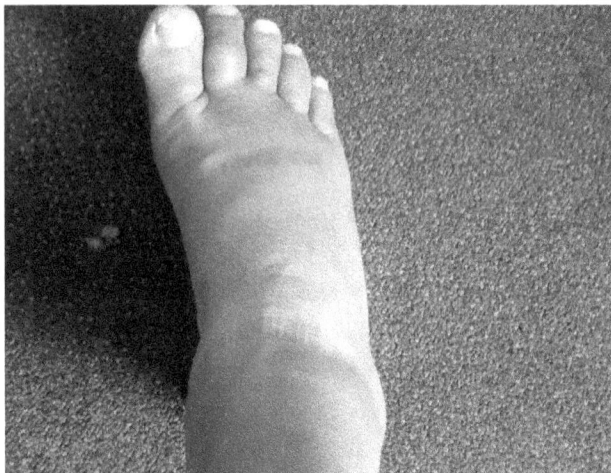

www.ingramcontent.com/pod-product-compliance
Lightning Source LLC
Chambersburg PA
CBHW022342280326
41934CB00006B/743